Sex-cription
The Natural Healing Power of 'SEX'

- Human Illnesses and Conditions you can cure naturally simply by having 'SEX'.

Mr. Paul M.

ISBN - 10: 1494746557
ISBN-13: 978-1494746551

DEDICATION

Dedicated to the honor of Nature and all the wonders it provides.

CONTENTS

Mr. Paul M.,

Mr. Paul M.,

ACKNOWLEDGMENTS

All glory to Almighty God and Father, the Author and Originator of all wonders.

1. INTRODUCTION

FACTS ABOUT SEX-CURES FROM STUDIES, RESEARCH, INTERVIEWS, SURVEYS, POLLS AND PERSONAL EXPERIENCES.

Sex-cription

Human illnesses that can be cured with 'SEX'

Sex is therapeutic when done right and can bring some emotional, psychological and even physical healing to the human person. It's true a lot of diseases including sexually transmitted diseases can be contacted through sex but little or nothing is seldom said about the immense and tremendous benefits of sex to the human body. Women especially, reap more benefits from the natural healing powers that come from sex more than men. Surprisingly, Mother Nature, the ultimate healer/physician has already diagnosed certain human illnesses/conditions and has prescribed sex for the cure. From arousal to foreplay to actual sex and to orgasm (a.k.a the big 'O'), amazing things happen within the inside and even the outside of the human body.

Both men and women share in the emotional and psychological healing benefit of sex but women receive more physical healing benefits from having sex with men. Of course the orgasm that comes from sex accounts for some of the emotional healing properties of sex but for a woman to have most physical healing from sex, it has to be with a man since the male spermatozoa deposited and absorbed by a woman's vagina amazingly contains certain natural ingredients designed to physically cure some illnesses/conditions within her body. Sound too good to be true, right? Don't just take my word for it.

I am pretty sure you've heard or used the phrase 'make up sex'. That common phrase alone suggests to you that sex has some emotional healing powers or ingredients that come with capable of healing both partners and thereby restoring the bond of their relationship and love. Sometimes couples get in each others faces, they argue hard, get mad at each other, go on strike at each other and in some extreme cases fight each other. But it's very interesting to see that what follows after this quarrel is hot sex which bonds them together all the more by healing those emotional picks and strengthening their relationship. That's why it's not very wise to get in between couples when they're having misunderstanding or trying to side for one against the other because once they have their make up sex, you will find yourself isolated.

Of course it's not every sex that brings healing to the body. By sex here I mean a consensual sex between a man and a woman without any force or coercion. Sex by rape (forced sex against the wish of the person) does not bring any healing to the person, rather it brings devastation. Sex abusive (taking advantage of a person sexually because of your authority over them) does not bring any kind of healing rather it brings anger, moodiness, withdrawal and lack of trust. For sex to bring all the emotional, psychological and physical healing properties it has, it has to be consensual, enjoyed and done regularly. Even a 'quickie' (one done in a hurry) has some benefits. Orgasm plays some role in some of the benefits we derive through sex. This means you can self-medicate yourself as often as you can and want to, even when your man is not available.

I guarantee you by the time you finish reading this book, you will start 'sex-capading', warming up your sheets again because sex is a powerful physician as old as the human existence. We stare him in face daily but never realized his healing capabilities. Not sexually active again or lost interest in sex? Identify what your problem is, might be from stress due to what's going on in your life now or from your past experience. May be you need to loose some weight, start eating right and exercising. If it might be caused by a medication condition, plan a trip to visit your physician. Whatever you need to do, do it, don't put it off. Do whatever you have to do to start warming the sheets again and often. This book will be your eye opener. Sex is a good thing, smell it, feel it, admire it, engage in it, taste it, it does amazing things to your brain, heart and body. OH MINE!!!

Let's get started and consider some of these human illnesses that can be cured with sex. It might surprise you and may be, it's time for you to start getting your 'grooves' on again.

So let's get down to it. As we said earlier, there are certain human illnesses and conditions that can be cured with sex. Both men and women benefit from sex in this regard but women reap more physical healing benefit from sex than their male counterparts. The following are some of these conditions/illnesses that having sex regularly and in the right way can help correct, cure and heal in the human body over time:

SEX AND STRESS, BETTER BLOOD PRESSURE:

Having sex could lower your stress and blood pressure. Studies has shown that great majority or record number of adults and even young adult undergo a lot of stress which emanates from the demands of everyday life and living. At certain age in life, we start taking on personal, family and even communal responsibilities. Stress can also come from our job, school works and a whole lot other undertakings apart from family responsibilities. Right before orgasming, women go into 'trance-like' state, says Kerner, activating parts of the brain that greatly help with stress-relief

Most of us will admit that extremely stressed-out and uptight folks could benefit from a nice under-the-bed-sheet activity. The pleasure from sex and orgasm relaxes you and calms your nerves. In a Scottish study, men and women were placed in stressful situations – such as speaking in public and doing math out loud - and told to keep record of their sexual activities. Afterwards they checked their blood pressure. Those who had recorded having intercourse responded better to stress than those who engaged in other sexual behaviors or abstained.

Another study found that diastolic blood pressure, which is the bottom number of your blood pressure, tends to be lower in people who live together and have sex often.

However, sex is not always included as a top stress management technique, despite all the physical and emotional benefits it provides. The fact and truth is, it should. Everyone should learn the stress management benefits of a healthy sex life. We should also learn how to get our grooves back if stress has put a damper on our libido.

Deep breathing relaxes your body, oxygenates your blood and reduces the stress you feel. Sense of touch is important because massage can be a great stress reliever. In fact, we need touch for our emotional health. Studies also shows that babies not touched enough can fail to thrive, and touch continues to be important into adulthood. Sexually active people tend to manage stress better, live longer and enjoy increased overall health.

The type of emotional intimacy that sex can supply is good for all of us. Endorphins released from sexual activity prevent stress effectively and sex is also able to release some other feel-good hormones. So when next you stressed out and need to relax, look no further than the bedroom.

SEX AND INSOMNIA/SLEEPLESSNESS:

You don't have to be a rocket scientist to understand how sex handles sleeplessness within the human body because whenever you have good sex that gives you orgasm, your muscles and nerves automatically relaxes due to the chemicals released by your brain and puts you in a sleep mode. Sleep of course helps recovery. When next you are experiencing sleeplessness which could be caused by a whole lot of issues, get your freak on under the blanket. It turns out that prolactin, the chemical released during orgasms also promotes sleep. After orgasm, the prolactin is released which is responsible for feeling of relaxation and sleepiness – says Sheenie Ambardar MD, a psychiatrist in West Hollywood CA. Prolactin level found to be naturally high when we sleep and because it's released after orgasm, we're put to sleep. No wonder after having one of those hot sex and exploding in one of them eye-curling orgasms, you body is put in a sleep mode for the next couple of hours.

However it's not any type of sex that will put your body in a sleep mode, it has to be enjoyed which culminates in at least one orgasm. More orgasms, more dose of sleeping pills. Orgasm releases the endorphin that calms your nerves, body and muscles, thereby creating an induced fatigue which in turn puts your body in sleep mode. So, any trouble hitting the hay? Forget pharmaceuticals, shut the bedroom door and dim the lights, whatever is it that gets you in the mood because sex is a natural dose/prescription for sleeplessness.

Both men and women experience the same sleeping mode effect of sex after experiencing orgasm. The sleep is deep, the rest is refreshing and rejuvenating. You want to do it over and over again but don't forget to set your alarm clock so you won't be late for work, office or miss that serious appointment.

SEX AND BEAUTY:

An orgasm is one of the healthiest things you can give to yourself everyday. It should be included in your routine along with brushing your teeth and washing your hair. So how does the orgasm from sex enhance your beauty? Check it out. Read ahead and find out how you can instantly improve your complexion by taking this advice to heart.

Sex makes your skin glow:

No need applying extra bronzer. Turns out the 'sex glow' is real. It's true – sex gives your skin a heavenly glow. Having sex improves oxygenation of the blood, blood circulation, which helps to pump oxygen to your skin and make it brighter. It also helps to eliminate toxins and can actually make your lips a little fuller. The effects of sex can do wonders to your complexion.

Ever heard of the phrase 'SEX-GLOW' before? It's real. No need for pore cleansers: Sex will do the trick, depending on how hot and heavy things are getting. By sweating during sex, you're actually giving your body a free facial. The sweat will clean from your pores the dirt, grime, and makeup residue you miss when you cleanse your face during the day. What follows after that? The amazing 'sex-glow'

So forget slapping on the latest retinol cream, sex can cure your dull skin, regular lovemaking causes more blood to rush through the body, revving up women's age-fighting elastin fibers. Outcome? Much tighter, fresher skin with an alluring after glow sex.

Sex can control acne:

Poor circulation can cause acne, dark spots and other skin diseases. Having sex regularly will accelerate circulation, balance your metabolism which will translate to a smooth delicate skin. Just as with people who exercise, having sex reduces your hormone levels and balances them out. The result? Clearer-looking skin, along with healthier hair! Sex also plays a role in prevention and treatment of skin disease.

Sex slows the aging process:

Hard to believe? Well bet'. Getting busy could set your clock back a few years as far as your appearance is concerned. As you have sex, you are boosting collagen production, which staves off age spots and sagging

Sex ward off wrinkles too:

Remember we said having sex boosts collagen production? That means it helps to keep you wrinkle-free in the process! Especially for those stressed-filled workweeks, we can't think of any facial mask that works as well as sex does for your skin.

Sex maintains the fountain of youthfulness:

We already told you that having sex will make you look and feel younger, but there is proof that others will notice too! A study was done on sex and youth a few years back to prove this point. In a span of 10 years, 3,500 men and women, both those who had sex regularly and those who didn't, were put on one side of a two-way mirror, where participants on the other side had to guess their age. The group that had an active sex life had their age underestimated by seven to 12 years, while some thought the group that only had sex infrequently actually looked older!

Sex strengthens your nails:

The same hormones that are released to make your skin glow will also keep your nails strong, especially during pregnancy, says Fulbright.

Sex hydrates your skin:

No, this doesn't mean you can replace your eight glasses of water with eight hours of sex, but having sex will keep your skin hydrated. Since it improves circulation, the blood will circulate around your body more efficiently, giving your skin the moisture it needs to stay healthy. This means no chapped lips and flaky dry skin any more.

Sex and Urinary Incontinence:

Let's understand urinary incontinence first. Urinary Incontinence is also known as 'loss of bladder control' or 'urinary leakage.' UI is when urine leaks out before you can get to a bathroom. If you have UI, you are not alone. Millions of women have this problem, especially as they get older.

Some women may lose a few drops of urine when they cough or laugh. Others may feel a sudden urge to urinate and cannot control it. Urine loss can also occur during sexual activity and can cause great emotional distress.

Causes of urinary incontinence: UI is usually caused by problems with muscles and nerves that help to hold or pass urine.

Urine is stored in the bladder. It leaves the body through a tube that is connected to the bladder called the urethra. Look at the images below to see how this process works.

Muscles in the wall of the bladder contract to force urine out through the urethra. At the same time, sphincter (ss-FINK-ter) muscles around the urethra relax to let the urine pass out of the body.

Incontinence happens if the bladder muscles suddenly contract or the sphincter muscles are not strong enough to hold back urine.

UI is twice as common in women as in men. Pregnancy, childbirth, and menopause are major reasons why. But both women and men can become incontinent from brain injury, birth defects, stroke, diabetes, multiple sclerosis, and physical changes associated with aging.

Pregnancy — Unborn babies push down on the bladder, urethra (tube that you urinate from), and pelvic floor muscles. This pressure may weaken the pelvic floor support and lead to leaks or problems passing urine.

- **Childbirth** — Many women leak urine after giving birth. Labor and vaginal birth can weaken pelvic floor support and damage nerves that control the bladder. Most problems with bladder control during pregnancy and childbirth go away after the muscles have time to heal. Talk to your doctor if you still have bladder problems 6 weeks after childbirth.

- **Menopause** — Some women have bladder control problems after they stop having periods. After menopause, the body stops making the female hormone estrogen. Some experts think this loss of estrogen weakens the urethral tissue.

Other causes of UI that can affect women and men are:

- **Constipation** — Problems with bladder control can happen to people with long-term (chronic) constipation.

- **Medicines** — UI may be a side effect of medicines such as diuretics ("water pills" used to treat heart failure, liver cirrhosis, hypertension, and certain kidney diseases). Hormone replacement has been shown to cause worsening UI.

- **Caffeine and alcohol** — Drinks with caffeine, such as coffee or soda, cause the bladder to fill quickly and sometimes leak.

- **Infection** — Infections of the urinary tract and bladder may cause incontinence for a short time. Bladder control returns when the illness goes away.

- **Nerve damage** — Damaged nerves may send signals to the bladder at the wrong time, or not at all. Trauma or diseases such as diabetes and multiple sclerosis can cause nerve damage. Nerves may also become damaged during childbirth.

- **Excess weight** — Being overweight is also known to put pressure on the bladder and make incontinence worse.

- **Stress incontinence** – Leakage happens with coughing, sneezing, exercising, laughing, lifting heavy things, and other movements that put pressure on the bladder. This is the most common type of incontinence in women. It is often caused by physical changes from pregnancy, childbirth, and menopause. It can be treated and sometimes cured.

- **Urge incontinence** – This is sometimes called "overactive bladder." Leakage usually happens after a strong, sudden urge to urinate. This may occur when you don't expect it, such as during sleep, after drinking water, or when you hear or touch running water.

- **Functional incontinence** – People with this type of incontinence may have problems thinking, moving, or speaking that keep them from reaching a toilet. For example, a person with Alzheimer's disease may not plan a trip to the bathroom in time to urinate. A person in a wheelchair may be unable to get to a toilet in time.

- **Overflow incontinence** – Urine leakage happens because the bladder doesn't empty completely. Overflow incontinence is less common in women.

- **Mixed incontinence** – This is 2 or more types of incontinence together (usually stress and urge incontinence).

- **Transient incontinence** – Urine leakage happens for a short time due to an illness (such as a bladder infection or pregnancy). The leaking stops when the illness is treated.

So how does sex help with urinary incontinence especially in women who stand the higher risk than men? About 30% of women will experience urinary incontinence in the cause of their life time. Regular sexual intercourse help strengthen the pelvic floor which controls the release of urine. Older women receive the greatest benefit: they can simply flex these sensitive muscles to avoid accidental leakage. Stronger pelvic muscles equal a better working urinary system.

For women, doing pelvic floor muscle exercise called Kegels may mean more pleasure, and as a perk, less chance of incontinence later in life. To do basic kegel exercise, tighten the muscles of your pelvic floor as if you're trying to stop the flow of urine. Count to 'three', then release. Repeat as often as necessary. For younger women, and indeed everyone, it's about time to start exercising those pelvic floor muscles by simply warming up the sheets and adding some kegel exercise.

SEX AND MIGRAINES:

The blinding pain and nausea of migraines may rule out intercourse, but science suggests sex cures away some of its pain. According to a 2001 study published in Headache, women who have intercourse while having a migraine lessened their pain by 30%, while 17.5% completely eliminated all migraine pains. With migraine, the serotonin released during orgasm causes a constriction of the dilated blood vessels in the brain. Clotted blood vessels most commonly were the cause of migraine.

The endorphin released during orgasm resembles morphine that can help ease annoying headaches, strained back or head-pounder – says Meston, PhD, Director of Sexual Psychophysiology Laboratory at the University of Texas, Austin. The increase in endorphin lasts for an estimated one to three hours. So you could have benefits from sex much longer than you might think. Studies conducted at Southern Illinois University found that half of female migraine sufferers reported relief after climaxing. Next time your head pounds with annoying migraine headache reach for your man and if he's not around, self-medicate and treat yourself to some solo sex ladies. As long as you hit the peak, masturbating will have the same soothing effect.

So next time you have migraines, save the pharmaceuticals for the next day, and instead of using that as an excuse to turn your back against your man facing the wall, reach towards him and get enough dose of sex to medicate your condition. Sex itself may be the relief or cure you desperately seek and need for that migraine headache.

SEX AND COMMON COLD:

Running nose, sneezing and wheezing, nothing is pretty about those at all. Want to combat the sniffles? Newsweek report sex can cure even the common cold. It works by raising immunoglobin A (a.k.a IgA) during intercourse, an important anti-body that helps fight the virus that causes the common cold. According to researchers at the Wilkes University, in Pennsylvania, these anti-bodies help combat disease and keep the body safe from colds and flu. Save up your sick days and swap those for your sex days baby.

SEX AND OUT-OF-CONTROL MENSTRUAL PERIOD:

Sex can give women lighter periods and fewer cramps. Women who has sex at least once a week can also reap the benefits of period regularity. Women who are intimate experience less erratic period. It does not work during a woman's period, you've got to get your time in before the period actually starts. Women's uterus contracts during orgasm, in which process it rids body of cramp-causing compounds. The increased number of contractions can also help expel blood and tissue more quickly helping to end your period faster. Sex during menstrual periods may not sound very appetizing due to worries about the bloody mess that will definitely occur. If your man does not hesitate, spread colored towel on a water-proof bed cover and stick with the missionary position.

Advice: Women-related health problems can be cured by sex but don't use it as an excuse to forgo healthy eating and a trip to the doctor. Sex can offer an easy fix, but it isn't the cure-all for all ailments.

SEX AND IMMUNE SYSTEM:

The good news is, sex is definitely good for you, at least in moderation. Psychologists prove that the immune systems of people who have sex once or twice a week receives significant boost. Scientists evaluate how robust our immune systems are measuring levels of immunoglobulin A, an antigen found in saliva and mucosal linings. This substance called the IgA, is the first line of defense against colds and flu. An important role of IgA is that it binds to pathogens at all points of entry to the body, and then calls on the immune system to destroy them.

In a study made to measure amounts of IgA in people who had sex and those who abstain from it, results showed that participants who had sex less than once a week had a small increase in IgA over those who abstained completely. Those who had one or two sexual encounters each week had a 30% rise. Unfortunately, people who had very frequent sex (three times a week or more) had lower IgA levels even than the abstainers.

Similar studies was conducted at Wikes University to prove that having sex once or twice a week has been linked with higher levels of an antibody previously referred to as Immunoglobin A, or IgA, which can protect you from getting cold and other infections. In the study, 112 students kept record of how often they had sex, providing saliva samples for the study. Those who had sex once or twice a week had higher levels of IgA than other students.

The high levels of IgA in volunteers who had moderately frequent sex are easy to understand. Sexually active people may be exposed to many more infectious agents than sexually non-active people may. The immune system may respond to these foreign antigens by producing and releasing more IgA. On the other hand, why there was no IgA rise in the most sexually active group, is not clear. So, want to boost your immune system? In addition to everything else you do to boost your immune system, don't forget to get your groove on.

SEX AND WEIGHT LOSS ('Sexercise'):

Depending on how intense, long or heavy the sexual intercourse is, sex can surprisingly help you burn more calories than you think. Some studies shows that thirty minutes of sex can burn up to 85 calories or more. It may not sound like much but it adds it up, especially if you have sex more often: 42 half-hour sessions will burn 3,570 calories, more than enough to loose a pound. Doubling up, you could drop that pound in 21 hour-long sessions. Sex is a great mode of exercise; though it takes both physical and psychological work to do it well.

How much calories sex is worth for a woman, studies did not confirm. This is because a woman's energy expenditure during sex is so variable. Some calorie-expenditure charts say that for the average 145-pound American lady, 20 minutes of moderate sex burns about 93 calories, more than a 20-minute stroll or leisurely cycling, about as much as a double tennis match.

SEX AND PROSTRATE CANCER IN MEN:

Studies had found out men with frequent ejaculations, up to 22 or more each month have the chances of prostate cancer being unlikely, especially if they started doing so in their 20's, may lower that risk of getting prostate cancer later on in their lives.

A published study in the Journal of American Medical Association discovered that men who had 21 or more ejaculations a month were less likely to get prostate cancer than those who had 4 – 7 per month.

However, there is no solid proof from the study that ejaculation is the only factor that matter when it comes to the odds of some men developing prostate cancer down the road as they age. The finding though is still taken into consideration and still holds.

SEX AND MEN'S HEART HEALTH:

In 2008 study published in the Journal of American College of Cardiology, erectile dysfunction (a.k.a E.D) is linked to poor cardio-vascular health. 2,300 men were studied and it was found that those with E.D had a 58% chance risk of coronary heart disease. There may be other causes though. Strong erection equals strong heart health. Sexually active life could ward of the risk of heart attack in for men. Studies have shown that sex is a great way to raise your heart rate and help keep estrogen and testosterone levels in balance. Low level on either of those chemicals in the body can put you at risk of developing an osteoporosis and even heart attack. So if you are a man and happen to observe your 'Mr. P' stays slump and soft especially when situation calls it for action to be up, hard and running, book and emergency appointment with your physician.

SEX AND BODY SHAPE/TONE:

Sex gives you more toned body, it's also a cardio exercise which can help you burn somewhere from 85 – 250 calories depending on the length of the fest. A quickie will burn fewer calories than all night long pleasure fest says Meston. Different parts of the body are worked out during sex. In fact cardiologists compared sexual activities to a modest workout on a treadmill as stated/published in an American Journal of Cardiology. You will also be squeezing in some sculpting: your abs and some muscles in your back, butt, thighs get a good workout as you thrust during sex. Depending on the intensity and endurance, partners sweat during sex, evidence that calories are being burnt. The sweat in turn cleanses your skin pores resulting in the famous 'sex-glow'.

SEX AND INCREASED BLOOD FLOW:

The heart start beating faster the moment we get excited and aroused about having sex, and blood start pumping at a faster rate, blood flow to our brain increases, these combine to result in better performance, increased oxygen supply to the body organs, thereby getting the system rid of old and waste substances. Sex cleanses the system.

SEX AND HEALTHY SPERM:

Several research and studies has shown that men who have frequent sex have relatively higher volumes of semen and increased sperm count compared to those who have infrequent sex. This is an exciting news for ladies since research has proved that the absorption of semen by a female body helps her fight depression, boost their energy and also can help them have smoother delivery as in the case with pregnant mothers.

SEX AND YOUR CAVITIES:

Men semen is chock-full of zinc, calcium and other tooth decay-fighting minerals that benefit women when their bodies absorb the semen from the men. It does not by any means replace your usual trips to your dentist but having extra doses of these minerals from male semen can't hurt.

SEX BOOSTS YOUR LIBIDO:

Sex boost your libido like a wild fire. All you need is to experience the sensational pleasure of orgasm, and it will automatically trigger a chain like reaction in your system because e your body will crave to experience this pleasure more often which of course results in an increased libido in both men and women. The more orgasm you experience the more your body will crave for it and the more sex you would want to have. Think your libido is not where it's supposed to be, get with the right partner or the right frame of mind to help you experience an orgasmic pleasure, the key to that engine that will get the chain reaction of an amazing libido started within your system.

SEX AND PAIN:

Talk of natural pain-killer for real. You can choose to save money on aspirins and use the natural prescription of orgasm to reduce or even eliminate your pains. So, aspirin or orgasm? Make your own choice. Study has shown that orgasm can block pain, yep! That's right, and you heard it loud and clear. We've said that already earlier. Endorphins released during orgasm act as morphine, pain-killer that can block chronic back and leg pains, can reduce menstrual cramps, arthritis pain and in some cases, even headaches including the annoying migraines.

SEX AND INTIMACY:

Sex boosts your intimacy with your partner. Study and research has shown that the more sexually active couples are towards each other, the more intimate they are compared to those with infrequent sex lives. The quarrel between sexually intimate active couples who have sex more frequently does not last as compared to those who are not very sexually active and frequent towards each other. This is where the magic of the make up sex works wonders in the life of a couple. So to increase intimacy with your partner, you've got to start warming each other up more often and very frequently too. If you're loosing your sexual appetite on your partner, try to identify the cause, discuss it together, seek help either from a friend or professional, and do whatever necessary to get connected again. Once that happens, don't ever put any type of hold on your sexual lives again.

SEX STRENGTHENS BOND:

Oxytocin is a hormone released by the brain during orgasm, it's also known as the 'the love hormone' – a bonding chemical. The release of this chemical helps people in building trust and in bonding with one another. The more sex a couple has, the more Oxytocin is released in their brain and by default, the more bonded they feel. Oxytocin also increases the feeling of generosity towards and between couples.

SEX AND SELF-ESTEEM:

There's good sex and equally there is great sex, the difference lies in self-esteem. Having great sex, ability to orgasm and give your partner orgasm each time you warm up under the sheets, actually boost your self-esteem and self-confidence. Not experiencing sex the way you should. Try figuring out what the problem is. You may need to start going to the gym, exercising, eating right or adjusting your wardrobe to provoke more sensual feelings in your partner towards you. In all and all, active and fulfilled sex life will definitely boost your self-esteem and confidence, you feel like taking on the world, it empowers you. We all know that experiencing orgasm is the crave of every sexually man and woman, the core of human pleasure which eludes many men and women. Your ability to be in touch with it makes you feel good about yourself and can affect your sense of self-esteem.

Studies and survey had suggested that when a woman is very sexually active and satisfied, it boost her self esteem and the way she feels about herself. But when a woman's sexual life is very passive and unsatisfying, it directly affects her sense of personal self esteem which may cause withdrawal, loneliness and some cases insecure. Same applies to men. When a man sexual is sexually active and knows how to hold it down in the bedroom, it really boosts his confidence and confidence plays a vital role in one's sense of personal self-esteem.

There you have it. There may be more health benefits of sex, as research, studies and surveys continue, but these are a few physical healing benefits we can get from sex. As you can see women benefit more physically from having sexual intercourse than men do. Please do not replace this with your normal healthy lifestyle; eating right, exercising and visit to your doctor. Sex benefit is as part of the family not in isolation.

CONCLUSSION

Nature has equipped the human body so many amazing capabilities to repair itself, fight germs and diseases, cure itself and adapt to the changing tune of the human environments. Excitingly we discovered sexual activities as one of those natural prescriptions with some wonderful ingredients that posses a healing power. Best of all, it's free and within the reach of every human person. You don't need a credit card or bank account, you don't need permission from anyone in other for you to get aroused or stimulated. If your partner is not available, you can self-medicate, treating yourself to a solo-sex and experience an orgasm which unlocks some of these healing properties. So what are you waiting for? Time to get started if you have not already.

Remember, sexual healing is a generic drug with universal label and you too can always prescribe it to someone else. However, for you to reap the full amazing benefits of sex, it has to be frequent and in a committed relationship. 'Quickies', casual sex, masturbation, can help us reap some of these benefits since you can stimulate and orgasm from them. But the immense full healing potential is experienced, especially for women, when it's done through intercourse between a man and a woman. Nature has endowed the male semen with some amazing ingredients such that when absorbed by the female body through vagina, these ingredients does amazing things inside the female body which science has proved and confirmed. This is why 'Sex-cription' is the newest generic drug in the market today.